In Defense of
SUGAR

The Sweet Truth about the Diet Industry's Latest Evil

By: Joey Lott

joeylotthealth.com

ISBN: 1518666817
ISBN-13: 978-1518666810

Table of Contents

Wrongly Accused

Just as the title suggests, this book is in defense of sugar, the much-maligned nutrient that is absolutely essential for human health. It *is* essential, but if you believe the hype, you'd believe that sugar is the work of the devil, created solely to tempt you and lead you to an early grave. But the hype is just that: hype. It's not the truth. It is, at best, a much-distorted misrepresentation of a small number of biased studies. At its worst, it is a fear-based, ideologically driven lie that, when believed, may lead to unnecessary suffering and ill health. And *that* is why I have written this book—to expose the lie and to help you free yourself from the fear and hysteria surrounding sugar.

In Defense of Sugar is titled as so precisely because sugar has been put on trial without any defense. The anti-sugar cult got a major shot in the arm in 1972 with the publication of John Yudkin's *Pure, White, and Deadly*. It continued to gain momentum with works such as Nancy Appleton's *Lick the Sugar Habit* and William Dufty's *Sugar Blues* just a handful of years later. But anti-sugarism only came into fashion in the past decade or so with the increasing influence of so-called ancestral (Paleo) diets and other low-carbohydrate dietary religions. Robert Lustig's popular video *Sugar: The Bitter Truth* and his book *Fat Chance* helped to foment the movement. Ever since then, there seems to be an all-out crusade against sugar as evidenced by the extreme popularity of

Sarah Wilson's *I Quit Sugar* and her eight-week program that challenges people to ditch the sugar.

Now, of course, if there really was credible evidence that sugar is such a bad thing, then I'd be all for anti-sugar advocacy. Granted, I wouldn't be in favor of attempts to legislate sugar, as is happening in various places around the globe now (e.g., taxes or outright bans on certain sugar-sweetened products), but rather for providing *information* to people. Yet, there's a difference between honest information and fearmongering that borders on the religious. And it is the latter that we are seeing a great deal of, by and large not backed up with credible evidence. We can volley wild claims and sensationalistic statements such as "sugar causes cancer" and "Alzheimer's is a sugar disease," but those types of debates lack substance. If we are merely going to offer up unsubstantiated claims or make claims based on poor or highly distorted evidence, then I could claim that oxygen causes cancer or that drinking water will kill you—incidentally, both claims are marginally true if distorted enough. But instead of throwing around such statements, I think it is better if we look at the evidence and see if it backs up the claims or not.

I began to research the peer-reviewed primary literature on the subject of sugar and health. I wanted to know if the claims had any credible evidence to back them and what I found was that the claims are unsubstantiated. In fact, the actual science paints a very different picture than what most anti-sugarists would have us believe. Far from being "pure, white, and deadly," it would seem that sugar is actually vital for human life. Granted, it *is* possible to convert non-carbohydrate sources into sugar, as necessarily happens on low-carbohydrate diets. But whether we obtain sugar from fruit and white sugar or indirectly from beef and coconut oil, our bodies do require sugar. The overly simplistic notion that sugar is inherently unhealthy or that some dietary sources of sugar are necessarily worse than others *for all people, all the time* turns out to be rather absurd. Can sugar be harmful in excess? Potentially. But then again, the same is true of water.

So I present to you a defense of sugar in which we will look at the actual science of human metabolism and the role that sugar plays. We will also look at some of the most common claims made by the anti-sugarists, and we'll scrutinize them to see if they hold up or not.

Before we get to the defense of sugar, however, I have to make a confession to you. Lest you believe that I am some "shill for the sugar industry" (and I thought *I* was paranoid!), I should confess to you that I was *terrified* of sugar for a good decade. I'm not exaggerating, either. I was genuinely scared of sugar. Being terrified of any food now seems absurd to me, but I had, at one time, bought into the anti-sugar propaganda, and I literally avoided all refined sugar for a decade. I wouldn't even *touch* it. Yes, I had some rather severe anxiety problems that extended well beyond food. Not only did I avoid all refined sugar but also all concentrated sugar sources such as honey and maple syrup. As I went further and further down the rabbit hole, I eventually found myself eliminating dried fruit, then fresh fruit, and finally even starchy carbohydrates.

The reason I feel I should make this confession is that, after a decade of avoiding sugar, and especially after a year of very low-carbohydrate dieting, I think it is hard to make the argument that I am simply addicted to sugar as many anti-sugarists will often say to attempt to dismiss any pro-balance arguments. Not only did I avoid it, but I had absolutely no desire for it. And, in fact, even now, after I have eaten sugar therapeutically in exceptionally large amounts, eating an average of a *pound* of granulated cane sugar *every day* for a year, I still have no cravings for sugar. I don't particularly like the taste of overly sweet foods, although I do quite like orange juice with all of its fructose goodness! In general, my feeling about sugar is that I can take it or leave it from a taste standpoint. I can state without any hesitation that my health is vastly superior when I include adequate sugar in my diet. That doesn't necessarily require eating large amounts of refined sugar, but neither does it preclude eating large amounts of refined sugar.

My own experience is merely what gets called an n=1 experiment. However, it turns out that I am not the only one. There are lots of people whose health is best when they include adequate amounts of sugar in their diets. That doesn't mean that everyone will always feel best when eating lots of sugar, but it certainly does call into question the popular sentiment that sugar is the root of all evil. And when looking into the actual science, it turns out that there's pretty good reason why people often feel better when eating adequate sugar, especially in the context of a nutrient-replete diet. That's because, in general, human bodies are designed to be able to handle lots of sugar. In fact, sugar is the preferred source of energy for many processes in the body.

On the other hand, when looking into the science, it starts to become clear why some people sometimes feel better when they eliminate sugar, at least temporarily. What the science suggests isn't so much that sugar is the problem, but that there may be metabolic complications that prevent some people from efficiently processing sugar. Since the body requires sugar to fuel various processes, being inefficient in handling sugar is hazardous. And while eliminating sugar may reduce the symptoms associated with metabolic complications, it isn't likely to do anything to repair the problem. So my own research strongly suggests that how well a person can metabolize sugar denotes good health, and if there are problems, then eliminating sugar isn't likely to be the ideal solution. But don't take my word for it. Let's look into the matter.

Sugar Isn't Merely Empty Calories

One of the ways in which sugar is often derided is with statements such as, "Sugar is nothing more than empty calories." These sorts of statements have been repeated often enough that many of us simply accept them as truth. But if we stop and look a little more closely, we may see that the statement is actually ridiculous. After all, what would make a calorie "empty"? The statement implies that the calories from sugar are somehow deficient in some fashion, whereas, in fact, a calorie from sugar is a calorie, and that calorie can be used to fuel essential processes in the body.

The simple reality is that we *need* calories. Not only that, but we need a *lot* of calories. We need *thousands* of calories every day. In fact, as I have detailed in other books, most of us need far more calories than we've been led to believe by the diet-obsessed culture in which we live. Most adults need somewhere between 2500 and 3500 calories every day on average, and the more active people are, the more the more calories they need.

Calories are so important that the lead researcher in the Minnesota Starvation Experiment, Ancel Keys, observed that calories alone were the key determinant in recovery from starvation. If calories were not sufficient (in his estimation, 4000 calories a day were required for recovery after 6 months of eating 1600 calories a day), then the composition of the diet (protein, carbohydrate, fat, and other nutrients such as vitamins and minerals) was of little consequence. In other words, the popular disdain for calories and the popular sentiment that seeks to *avoid* calories may be horribly misguided, and because many of us are still at least partially under the spell of that sort of thinking, we may overlook the insanity of a statement such as, "Sugar is nothing more than empty calories."

The truth is that sugar is one of the supreme sources of essential nutrition. I am not suggesting that eating nothing apart from refined sugar is an ideal diet. However, sugar, whether from white sugar or fruit or any other source, provides essential energy (calories) in an easily digested format. Every cell in your body needs energy, and those "empty calories" in sugar turn out to be not so empty. Instead, they're complete sources of energy.

When people suggest that sugar provides "empty calories," what they *really* mean to say is that sugar provides calories, which are essential, but depending on the form of sugar (e.g., refined, white sugar), it may not provide many *other* nutrients, which is a valid criticism, of course. As I suggested, eating a diet composed exclusively of white sugar would lead to nutrient deficiencies. So it is important to eat a diet that includes a full complement of nutrients. To slander sugar because it does not provide *complete* nutrition is shortsighted because, in fact, *no* food (except, perhaps, milk) can provide complete nutrition. You would eventually wind up with nutrient deficiencies if you ate nothing except meat, nothing but broccoli, or nothing but coconut. So by the same logic, we could call broccoli or meat "empty calories." It is nothing more than a propaganda technique, but if you truly question it, you can see that it is ridiculous.

Sugar, whether from white sugar, fruit, or any other source, provides at *least* one *essential* nutrient, which is the sugar itself. The human brain, on average, requires about 120 grams of sugar every day in order to function. In extreme situations, the brain can get by with less sugar, instead relying on ketones and/or lactate for approximately half of its energy requirements. No matter what, the brain *always* requires substantial sugar. If it is deprived of sugar even for a few minutes, that would be the end of you. And it is worth pointing out that, despite the claims to the contrary promoted by low-carb enthusiasts, the bulk of the evidence is that ketones are *stressful* for the body and used only when adequate sugar isn't available. For example, even in the context of a very low-carbohydrate diet, the body will actually convert protein to sugar in order to provide energy for the brain. To sustain ketosis, it is necessary to eat a low-carbohydrate *and* a low-protein diet in which the overwhelming majority of the calories come from fat. That strongly suggests that the body *prefers* sugar to the more stressful ketones. There's a reason why most of us would experience nausea when eating extremely small amounts of carbohydrates and protein while guzzling medium-chain triglyceride oil. It's because, generally speaking, our bodies strongly desire carbohydrates (i.e., sugar), and ketosis is not a preferred state.

More Addictive than Cocaine

One of the more sensationalistic claims leveled against sugar is that it is addictive. In fact, a popular statement is that "sugar is more addictive than cocaine and heroin." This is based, at least in part, on studies that have made the absurd comparison.[1] I write that it is an absurd comparison because it utterly defies the human experience.

Although the anti-sugarists are quick to advertise the results of any studies that support their thesis, they often do so in a manner that distorts the actual findings. For example, popular anti-sugarists such as Dr. Mark Hyman, Dr. Joe Mercola, and Dr. Terry Wahl have all published articles citing rat studies claiming that sugar is more addictive than cocaine or heroin. But none of them pointed out that the studies could easily be interpreted in many other ways. For example, one study gave rats a choice between Oreos or cocaine. The rats often, though not always, chose Oreos. But does that actually prove that Oreos are more addictive than cocaine? No, it does not. It merely demonstrates that in that context, some rats sometimes chose Oreos over cocaine. But guess what? Some humans, if given a choice between Oreos or cocaine, would choose Oreos while others would

---

[1] Lenoir et al. Intense Sweetness Surpasses Cocaine Reward. Public Library of Science. 2007; 2(8): e698.

choose cocaine. (I'd choose neither, frankly, but I'm not sure if that was really an option for the rats.) All it proves is that people make different choices sometimes. So maybe some rats just don't like cocaine? Maybe some of them really like Oreos? But so what?

The claim that sugar is more addictive than many drugs known to be highly addictive is the sort of thing that makes for good headlines. And people who want to believe in the anti-sugar message will latch on to these sorts of internet memes precisely because of their sensationalistic nature. I mean, if you are at a party and the conversation turns to sugar, rattling off something like, "Studies have found that sugar is more addictive than cocaine" can make you feel like you've got something important to say. It's an attention-grabber. And that's why that sort of nonsense gets kept alive, because bloggers and doctors who have built their reputations on hating sugar regurgitate anything that supports their cause. That doesn't make it true, however.

Other studies have looked at the brain activity involved in human participants shown food, or images of food, and then given food to eat. In one such study,[2] a group of 48 young women were shown a chocolate milkshake and then given the milkshake to eat. The researchers monitored brain activity in the young women during the process. What they observed was that areas of the brain associated with decision making were activated during the presentation of the milkshake. The researchers noticed that the women who had reported low levels of food cravings in general had significant activity occurring in a part of the brain that is associated with reward or satisfaction once they were given the milkshake, whereas the young women who reported having food cravings in general showed *less* activity in that part of the brain when compared to the first group. Because a similar pattern of reduced satisfaction brain activity is seen in some drug addictions, the researchers and anti-sugarists in particular have

---

[2] Gearhardt et al. The Neural Correlates of "Food Addiction." Archives of General Psychiatry. 2011; 68(8): 808-816.

concluded that food, and particularly sugar, must be addictive. At least it is for the handful of people who report food cravings.

But let's face it. These conclusions are bogus. Of course people can make *anything* into the object of an addiction. Heck, I used to be "addicted" to washing my hands. People can fixate on anything. So, yes, there may be some people who seem to have genuinely addictive and unhealthy relationships with sugar and start sneaking, hiding, bingeing, etc. But then again, there are people who have similar relationships with walking, cleaning, reading, and all kinds of things. And in general, it's *really* hard to argue that sugar is *inherently* as addictive as cocaine or heroin. I mean, I've seen the lines outside of methadone clinics. People have a *really* hard time giving up heroin and cocaine. They do *not* have the same difficulties with sugar. And the bottom line is that just because a rat chooses Oreos or hungry people aren't satisfied after eating doesn't prove *anything* about sugar. Think about it.

Anti-sugarists such as Dr. Mark Hyman claim that, just as one can't simply cut down on heroin or cocaine use, neither can one merely cut down on sugar intake. He claims (as do others) that one has to completely eliminate sugar from one's diet. Otherwise, the tiniest bit of sugar, just the same as the tiniest bit of heroin, will set off a massive binge. But this is pure propaganda that has no basis in reality. Just about everyone I have ever communicated with and every book or webpage I have read that provides accounts of people *reducing* (but not eliminating) sugar intake refutes this claim. In general, people are perfectly capable of reducing sugar intake. Most people are capable of eating a bite of a chocolate bar without feeling powerless as they inhale the whole thing at once. I am well aware that *some* people have trouble with this. I used to be one of them. For years I would regularly eat well beyond comfort and *still* desire more. But that is a different phenomenon entirely, having nothing whatsoever to do with sugar addiction. More likely it is a combination of being hungry [yes, even fat people] and psychological conditioning. And in my experience, when people are able to resolve the metabolic problems and psychological conditioning that lead to the phenomenon, all foods, including sugar, are desired and eaten without any signs of "addiction." Sugar is *not* the same as heroin or cocaine. People who claim otherwise are either completely delusional or they are blatantly lying.

The real kicker, however, is that the supposed signs of "food addiction" as seen in brain monitoring studies show up in response to *any* food.[3] In fact, the response shows up merely at the presentation of an *image* of food. Not surprisingly, the responses tend to be stronger in fatter people. I say that's not surprising because fat people are generally legitimately *hungrier*. That can be for a variety of reasons, and not all are understood. In some cases, cellular respiration is impaired. In some cases, the endogenous cannabinoid system is dysregulated, producing a chronic state of "the munchies." But the food is not addictive. Sugar is not addictive. There may simply be metabolic problems that lead some people to respond more strongly than others and to feel less satisfied than others. It is possible to make changes that will alleviate the problems, and those changes don't involve eliminating sugar. In fact, ironically, restriction is one of the things that can fuel metabolic imbalances that, in turn, create a strong desire for food.

The anti-sugarists are being awfully selective in their interpretation of the information. It's curious that they aren't so quick to ban or tax milk despite the fact that milk is a key ingredient in milkshakes. Nor are they calling for a ban on images of food despite the fact that images of food can produce the same "addictive" response in people. Though, I suppose those sentiments are sure to come forward sooner or later.

Moreover, what is being observed in these studies doesn't even make a strong case for addiction. Instead, it seems to me that what is being reported is that people respond to food. That really shouldn't be a surprise. After all, we need food, and we've

---

[3] Davids et al. Increased dorsolateral prefrontal cortex activation in obese children during observation of food stimuli. International Journal of Obesity. 2010; 34(1): 94-104.

presumably evolved over millions of years to have strong responses to food. Furthermore, in spite of the sensationalistic headlines claiming that "studies prove sugar is addictive," other levelheaded scientists and academics concur with my conclusion: there is no credible evidence that sugar is addictive.[4]

---

[4] Benton D. The plausibility of sugar addiction and its role in obesity and eating disorders. Clinical Nutrition. 2010; 29(3): 288-303.

Sugar Causes Diabetes

It would seem that most people have effectively accepted that sugar is the cause of diabetes (in this case we're mostly talking about type 2 diabetes). In fact, diabetes is one of the most common themes that comes up in any discussion of sugar. The truth is that no one knows for certain what causes diabetes. However, for reasons that we'll see shortly, there are much more likely suspects than sugar. Yet the simplicity of the claim that sugar causes diabetes appeals to many people, and as such, it is a popular, although mistaken, belief. Many of us make the mistake of believing that we can protect ourselves against diabetes by eliminating sugar from our diets. That may give us a sense of security and smugness, but it is a false sense of security simply because there is actually no evidence that sugar causes diabetes.

Diabetes was first reported approximately 3,500 years ago. It was noted that people suffering from the condition had excessive urination and that their urine was sweet. The urine attracted ants and other sugar-seeking insects. As a result, diabetes quickly became associated with sugar.

It is now thought that the loss of sugar in the urine of diabetics is due to either a lack of insulin (most common in cases of type 1 diabetes in which the pancreas no longer produces sufficient insulin) or insulin resistance in the cells. In either case, the blood sugar, glucose, that is normally used by cells cannot be properly taken up by them. Because elevated levels of blood sugar can produce problems, the body compensates by dumping the sugar into the urine. That is, of course, a problem because the cells aren't able to use the energy. As a result, diabetes was traditionally a death sentence in which the diabetic became fatigued and emaciated before dying.

Now, here's an interesting thing. For thousands of years, diabetics continued to lose sugar in their urine *even if* they virtually eliminated all sugar from their diets. There are accounts of doctors in the 1800s who monitored the sugar content of diabetic patients eating an exclusively meat-based diet and found that they continued to lose large amounts of sugar in the urine. For example, the celebrated English physician William Budd wrote an account of a woman who "in the intimate persuasion that an exclusive animal diet could alone cure her, had the courage to subject herself to it during nearly two months without deviating from it for a single day."[5] He reports that prior to undertaking the carnivorous diet, she was losing 27 grams of sugar per pint of urine. Although the carnivorous (very low-carbohydrate) diet initially reduced the sugar loss, it then began to rise again, eventually to 49 grams per pint! Why this should be so, of course, is not especially surprising to us today because it is now known that the body will convert proteins and fat to sugar to meet the body's energy needs. Of course, if insulin is not sufficient or if the cells are resistant to insulin, that glucose will not be used and instead will be dumped into the urine. And, it is also now known that low-carbohydrate diets tend to *increase* insulin resistance while high-carbohydrate diets *decrease* insulin resistance. So a woman who already has insulin-resistance symptoms is likely to start dumping *even more* sugar when she greatly reduces her carbohydrate intake.

What is curious, however, is that the low-sugar, low-carbohydrate diet continues to be prescribed to diabetics today.

---

[5] Braithwaite, William. The Retrospect of Medicine, Volume 37. Simpkin, Marshall, and Company. 1858.

Of course, a ketogenic diet may get around this obstacle of impaired oxidative respiration at the cellular level by forcing the body into using an alternate energy source: ketones. So for some diabetics, a ketogenic diet may act as a stopgap measure or as a survival strategy. However, it certainly is not a *cure*.

William Budd, the same who reported about the woman who continued to lose sugar in her urine after eating a low carbohydrate diet, also reported of a case in which, despite all his efforts, a diabetic patient was continuing to deteriorate rapidly. He made a decision, inspired by the work of a French physician who had seen success in diabetics by feeding them sugar, to put the man on a diet that included eight ounces of sucrose (white sugar) and six ounces of honey *every day*. The man quickly began to return to health. Budd does *not* report on the long-term outcome of this approach, and notably, the man did *not* cease to lose sugar in his urine, so I am not necessarily proposing that sugar feeding is always an appropriate treatment for diabetes. However, it certainly does pose a challenge to the notion that sugar is the cause of diabetes. Furthermore, another physician, George Corpe, also included a report in the same publication in which he treated a diabetic man with a diet consisting of sufficient fructose from sugar candy, honey, and sweet root vegetables. He had the man eliminate, or at least greatly reduce, starches from his diet with the idea being that glucose (the sugar in starch) eaten without sufficient fructose (as is found in white sugar, honey, and sweet root vegetables) may be poorly metabolized, whereas sufficient fructose may resolve the problem. Interestingly, Corpe reported that the man not only returned to health, but he *stopped losing sugar in his urine* with the dietary treatment prescribed.

Again, those are only two case studies, and in and of themselves, they don't prove anything. But they *do* challenge the common belief that sugar causes diabetes. And they are further backed by the fact that fructose has been used successfully in the long-term glycemic control of diabetics. A meta-analysis published in the American Diabetes Association's *Diabetes Care* journal concluded, after reviewing eighteen controlled feeding trials in which fructose was substituted for other carbohydrates, that the fructose substitution resulted in better blood sugar control.[6]

As already stated, diabetes is defined by the inability of the body to properly metabolize sugar. That *does not* mean that sugar causes diabetes. Rather, sugar control is a problem *because* of diabetes. In other words, people who claim that sugar causes diabetes likely have the cart before the horse.

What is curious to me is that in the conversation about diabetes, there is a great deal of focus on insulin and elevated sugar in the blood, but there is very little mention of the fact that one of the symptoms of diabetes is also *elevated free fatty acids*. And, when digging into the literature, it turns out that the significance of elevated free fatty acids may be anything but incidental.

Free fatty acids are, as the name suggests, the fatty acid building blocks of fats that have been broken apart into their unbound form. For example, when you eat food containing butter, that fat may get broken into individual fatty acids that include butyric acid, palmitic acid, oleic acid, stearic acid, and others. Or, through a process called "de novo lipogenesis," the body may synthesize new fatty acids. Those fatty acids may be used for various processes in the body, and they may be stored in fat cells. When the fat cells release fatty acids into the blood, those fatty acids are called free fatty acids.

Free fatty acids are secreted by the fat cells when the body is in need of energy that isn't being supplied by glucose (blood sugar). Despite the bickering that often occurs between pro-carbohydrate and anti-carbohydrate dietary cults, it would seem that a healthy human body is capable of using both glucose and free fatty acids largely interchangeably for most muscles, and that is a good thing. If the body has trouble metabolizing *either*, then it is in trouble. So in a healthy body, when glucose is present, it is used readily, and when free fatty acids are present, they are used

---

[6] Cozma et al. Effects of Fructose on Glycemic Control in Diabetes. Diabetes Care. 2012; 35(7): 1611-1620.

readily. There are some specialized organs that strongly prefer glucose, of course. For example, as noted earlier, the brain needs a lot of glucose. So glucose and free fatty acids are not entirely interchangeable in all cases, but most muscles should be able to use either form of energy.

The problem in diabetes seems to be that, not only is blood sugar elevated, but so are free fatty acid levels. And furthermore, there may be reason to suspect that the elevated free fatty acids may actually be *causing* the elevated blood sugar. Not many researchers seem to be investigating this angle, but those who are are revealing some important clues. For example, a paper from Temple University Hospital in Philadelphia [7] explains that elevated free fatty acid levels in the blood are found in cases of high body fat, insulin resistance, and type 2 diabetes, and that free fatty acids in the blood suppress the ability of cells to uptake blood sugar. In a more recent paper by the same author,[8] it was explained that not only do elevated free fatty acids in the blood likely produce insulin resistance (and type 2 diabetes in those who cannot compensate adequately), but they also activate inflammatory processes that may produce some of the symptoms of diabetes such as cardiovascular disease.

Other studies have suggested that when it comes to free fatty acids, they may not all be created equal. Some types may be benign or even beneficial while others may be harmful. Although many researchers and medical professionals (not to mention organizations such as the American Diabetes Association) have been quick to recommend that diabetics, and everyone else, should reduce or eliminate saturated fats and instead substitute polyunsaturated fats, it now seems that may have been very bad advice, indeed.

---

[7] Boden G. Free fatty acids, insulin resistance, and type 2 diabetes mellitus. Proceedings of the Association of American Physicians. 1999; 111(3): 241-248.

[8] Boden G. Effects of free fatty acids (FFA) on glucose metabolism. Experimental and Clinical Endocrinology and Diabetes. 2003; 111(3): 121-124.

Doctor Elliot Berry, MD, of the Hebrew University in Jerusalem published a paper[9] in which he observed that, despite the popular claims that polyunsaturated fat intake should protect against diabetes and a whole host of diseases, Israel, the country with the highest consumption of omega-6 polyunsaturated fats in the world, also has some of the highest rates of diabetes, cardiovascular disease, and other conditions supposed to be protected against by polyunsaturated fat. He concludes, as other researchers are now beginning to conclude, that polyunsaturated fat, and *particularly* omega-6 polyunsaturated fat may, in fact, be problematic.

In his paper, Berry suggests that the omega-3 to omega-6 fatty acid ratio may be significant and that adequate omega-3 intake from fish oils may offset some of the negatives of omega-6 fatty acid intake. He is not alone in this contention, of course. A number of studies have demonstrated the potential protective value of omega-3 fatty acids from fish oil in diets that otherwise include significant amounts of omega-6 fatty acids. However, as some authors from the National Institutes of Health concluded,[10] although omega-3 fatty acids can offset the negative effects of omega-6 fatty acids, the actual value of supplemental omega-3 fatty acids is largely null when omega-6 fatty acids are low enough in the diet. In other words, slamming down fistfuls of fish oil capsules may be a misguided approach to improving health. A better approach may be to simply eliminate highly polyunsaturated fat sources such as soy oil, corn oil, and canola oil from the diet.

Although a lot of research still demonstrates that omega-3 fatty acid supplementation can provide *some* potential benefits in the context of diabetes (as well as other disease conditions), much of that research is myopic. However, some research is starting to

---

[9] Berry EM. Are diets high in omega-6 polyunsaturated fatty acids unhealthy? European Heart Journal. 2001; 3(Supplement D): D37-D41.

[10] Hibbeln et al. Healthy intakes of n-3 and n-6 fatty acids. American Journal of Clinical Nutrition. 2006; 83(6): S1483-S1493.

come out that demonstrates the shortcomings of *all* polyunsaturated fats in excess. One such study[11] looked at the effects of feeding saturated fat versus a high omega-3 polyunsaturated fat diet to diabetic patients. What they found was that both diets resulted in an improvement in blood lipid markers. However, the *polyunsaturated* diet resulted in *worsening* blood sugar control when compared to the saturated fat diet.

To be clear, there is certainly no scientific consensus on this matter. However, it certainly seems *likely* that elevated free fatty acids, and *particularly* polyunsaturated free fatty acids from a diet that includes lots of seed oils and fats from grain-fed animals, may be strongly implicated in diabetes whereas sugar does *not* appear to be. That certainly does not mean that polyunsaturated fat is *always* the cause of type 2 diabetes, of course. But it does seem to be a likely candidate in many cases. Meanwhile, sugar *metabolism* is impaired as a result, and dietary sugar is wrongly blamed.

---

[11] Vessby et al. Polyunsaturated fatty acids may impair blood glucose control in type 2 diabetic patients. Diabetic Medicine. 2009; 9(2): 126-133.

Sugar Feeds Cancer Cells?

Another one of the common sensationalistic claims made by the anti-sugarists is that sugar feeds cancer cells. Now, technically, this seems to be a true statement. However, as it turns out, it's a loaded and misleading statement. Sure, sugar feeds cancer cells; it also feeds *the rest of the cells in your body*. That includes your brain cells, by the way. Sugar is an energy source—an *essential* energy source—for the human body.

The anti-sugarist stance in regard to cancer likely stems from observations made by the German biochemist Otto Warburg, the recipient of the 1931 Nobel Prize in Physiology. He was awarded the prize for his discoveries in cellular respiration with a particular interest in cancer cells. Warburg observed that "the prime cause of cancer is the replacement of the respiration of oxygen in normal body cells by a fermentation of sugar."

This observation could easily be misrepresented, and has been, to suggest that sugar is the prime cause of cancer. However, Warburg never claimed that sugar was the cause of cancer. In fact, he even explicitly cautioned against that misinterpretation, claiming that attempts to starve cancer cells by withholding dietary sugar would be a mistake. His observation was that in normal cells, sugar is oxidized, whereas in cancer cells, sugar is fermented anaerobically. Therefore, a more accurate way to restate the observation is that a lack of oxygen is what differentiates the processes of cancer cells versus non-cancer cells. Sugar is used by both types of cells, but the *way* in which the sugar is used differs. Some have stated that cancer may, in fact, be a last ditch effort of cells to produce energy when normal oxidative respiration is impaired.

A popular claim by anti-sugarists is that one way to cure cancer is to starve cancer cells of sugar. However, as should hopefully already be obvious, that may not be the best idea. Not only will the body produce sugar (glucose) even if dietary sugar is avoided, but there is also evidence that cancer cells may use amino acids to fuel tumor growth.[12] So simply eliminating sugar from one's diet will likely do nothing to starve cancer cells, at least no more than it will starve the rest of the cells in your body.

Now, there is *some* tentative evidence that demonstrates that ketones, which are an energy source produced from fat, may suppress both glucose *and* glutamine metabolism in *some* cells *sometimes*. Based on that, there is the *possibility* that an extreme ketogenic diet *may* have some therapeutic value in some cases of cancer. However, that is yet to be demonstrated in practice. And, furthermore, *even* if it has limited therapeutic value in some cases, it is certainly *not* true that a ketogenic diet is an effective prophylactic against cancer. Again, ketosis has *not* yet been demonstrated to actually have any practical application in the treatment of cancer. However, even if it does, it is important to maintain perspective. For example, chemotherapy has a track record of successfully treating cancer. Radiation treatment also has a successful track record. However, that does not mean that chemotherapy or radiation treatment should be used as prophylactics!

To date, no one knows definitively what causes cancer. However, the idea that sugar causes cancer is absurd. Sugar is an energy source for all cells—cancerous or not. The most promising therapies and preventions of cancer are those that seek

---

[12] Le et al. Glucose-independent glutamine metabolism via TCA cycling for proliferation and survival in B cells. Cell Metabolism. 2012; 15(1): 110-121.

to maintain healthy, oxidative cellular respiration, *not* those that seek to starve or go to war with the body. And with that in mind, it is interesting to note that research is now indicating that polyunsaturated fat may be one of the causes of impaired cellular respiration. For example, a 2013 study found that dietary intake of polyunsaturated fats may result in "cellular dysfunction and contribute to cancer risk and progression."[13] And, as we saw previously, the bulk of the evidence suggests that omega-6 fatty acids may be the primary culprits. Though omega-3 fatty acids may partially mediate the negative effects of omega-6 fatty acids, the most sensible thing to do, in light of research, is to reduce omega-6 fatty acid intake. It is at least plausible that cellular respiration may be able to resume normally in the absence of excessive polyunsaturated fat.

---

[13] Azrad et al. Current evidence linking polyunsaturated fatty acids with cancer risk and progression. Frontiers in Oncology. 2013; 3: 224.

Fructose

The majority of the anti-sugarists have become increasingly sophisticated and specific in their attacks on sugar. Many now concede that dietary glucose is likely not problematic in most cases. Glucose is a simple sugar, the main sugar found in the blood, and is used for cellular respiration. Glucose is what the body will produce from carbohydrates, protein, or fats to meet its energy needs. When glucose forms a complex sugar with other glucose molecules, it is called starch, and when it forms a complex sugar with fructose, it is called sucrose, which is what common white sugar is.

So while glucose is increasingly accepted, even among anti-sugarists (although many of them despise glucose all the same), *fructose* is now being labeled as the bad guy. Fructose, as we've already seen, occurs naturally in the complex sugar sucrose, in which each molecule of fructose is paired with a molecule of glucose in a bound form. As mentioned, white sugar is essentially pure sucrose. Maple syrup also contains sucrose as the primary sugar, and sucrose is found in varying amounts in fruits and vegetables. Fructose also occurs in an unbound form alongside unbound glucose and sometimes sucrose in honey, fruit, and some vegetables. In general, fructose tends to occur naturally in close to a 1-to-1 ratio with glucose. For example, sucrose is one fructose molecule to each glucose molecule. In honey, the ratio of unbound fructose to unbound glucose is often *approximately* 1-to-1 (some types of honey will have higher ratios than others). And in many fruits, the total ratio of fructose to glucose is close to 1-to-1, though some fruits are higher in fructose than others. For example, apples have a fructose to glucose ratio of about 3-to-1 (depending on the variety), and most pear varieties have about a 2-to-1 ratio. But in general, when eating *naturally occurring* sweet foods, the fructose to glucose ratio will be fairly close to 1-to-1. That does *not* mean that the average diet includes fructose and glucose in a 1-to-1 ratio. In fact, most diets involve *vastly* more glucose than fructose. That's because many foods contain glucose but *no* fructose. For example, starchy foods contain glucose only. So it is estimated that, on average, the ratio of the dietary intake of fructose to glucose is 1-to-5.

The main argument for why fructose is supposedly so bad for health is that it is metabolized differently than glucose. Fructose reportedly is absorbed *primarily* by the liver. Other organs and even muscles can reportedly process fructose as well, but the liver is said to have the greatest capacity in this regard. In the liver, approximately 50 percent of fructose is said to be converted into glucose, which by admission of anti-sugarists is not problematic. Another 25 percent is converted to lactate,[14] which may be used readily by the brain.[15] Approximately 20 percent is converted to glycogen, which is the essential energy storage format that the liver maintains in order to power the brain. The remainder of the fructose is converted to carbon dioxide or converted to the *saturated* fatty acid, palmitic acid. Of course, when we look at the facts in this way, it is difficult to see what all the fuss is about. Why is fructose said to be the bad guy if all that is happening is

---

[14] Dietze et al. Utilization of glucose and fructose in human liver and muscle. Internationale Zeitschrift für Vitamin- und Ernährungsforschung. Beiheft. 1976; 15: 31-43.

[15] Wyss et al. In vivo evidence for lactate as a neuronal energy source. Journal of Neuroscience. 2011; 31(20): 7477-7485.

that it gets converted to energy sources and a small amount of palmitic acid?

The reason that fructose is said to be so terrible is that in *extreme* feeding studies in which participants were given free fructose in great excess of what could ever be achieved through natural dietary means, the participants developed fatty deposits on their livers. But let's put this in perspective. One such study[16] fed 3.5 grams of free fructose per kilogram of body mass, which was estimated to be approximately 35 percent of total energy intake. Even though it is estimated that North American diets have doubled their fructose intake in the last half century, the average fructose intake of North Americans only accounts for 6 percent of total energy intake. And even at the upper levels of fructose intake, total fructose intake rarely accounts for more than 12 percent of energy intake. So this feeding study was using amounts of fructose that are six times what the average North American eats and three times what even the most dedicated fructophiles are eating. In addition to that, the participants were fed pure fructose, a substance that does not exist in isolation in the natural world. We also don't know what impacts may or may not have been attributed to the solvent residues and other impurities in the fructose provided in the study. So although the anti-sugarists are quick to use studies such as this one as evidence that fructose is dangerous, the reality is that all the study proves is that humans fed industrially produced free fructose at 35 percent of their energy intake may develop fatty deposits on their livers. That doesn't say *anything* about what natural fructose in more reasonable amounts (even at the extreme range of 12 percent energy intake) will or will not do. However, when we look at the studies that look at the effects of natural fructose intake in reasonable amounts, what we find is that there isn't much evidence of negative consequences.

---

[16] Le et al. Fructose overconsumption causes dyslipidemia and ectopic lipid deposition in healthy subjects with and without a family history of type 2 diabetes. American Journal of Clinical Nutrition. 2009; 89(6): 1760-1765.

Still, anti-sugar propaganda everywhere now claims that fructose causes non-alcoholic fatty liver disease (NAFLD), which, as the name suggests, is a condition in which the liver has lots of fatty deposits. What is the evidence? Well, as we've already seen, there really isn't any. The studies that demonstrate that fructose can produce fatty deposits involve extreme feeding of free fructose to the extent that is impossible to achieve with food. And furthermore, there are even studies that show that in terms of fructose from food, higher fructose intake is actually correlated with a *decreased* risk of developing NAFLD.[17]

Still, anti-sugarists claim that fructose depletes ATP (adenosine triphosphate, an important energy source in the human body) in the liver, which could *theoretically* produce liver problems like NAFLD. However, as usual, the only studies that demonstrate this phenomenon are those that use unnaturally high concentrations of free fructose, which is often *injected* into the subjects. These studies do show that large amounts of free fructose injected into the liver can deplete ATP. However, notably, the same thing does *not* happen when fructose is coupled with glucose. This is not surprising, of course, since one of the major benefits of sugar metabolism is the generation of large amounts of ATP. And frankly, if fructose was *that* toxic, early humans feasting on tropical fruits would have dropped dead before they could have produced the next generation.

Interestingly, as we saw earlier, research into the effects of fructose in diabetes has shown that replacing glucose with fructose in diabetics may actually improve blood sugar control. And we also read of two accounts of unconventional diabetes treatments in which the diabetics were fed sugar (and in one case starch was limited), which would have resulted in an increase in fructose consumption. In both cases, the diabetics experienced dramatic health improvements. I am not claiming that fructose

---

[17] Kanerva et al. Higher fructose intake is inversely associated with risk of non-alcoholic fatty liver disease in older Finnish adults. American Journal of Clinical Nutrition. 2014; 100(1): 1133-1138.

should always be used as a treatment for diabetes. However, this information does cast some doubt on the claims that fructose is such a bad thing.

A group of researchers at Yale University performed a study[18] in which they hoped to test whether the main defect in diabetes was due to insulin resistance per se or impaired cellular respiration. They fed the participants 75 grams of glucose and monitored the effects. They then fed the participants 75 grams of fructose and monitored the effects. What they found was that glucose failed to produce any improvement in cellular respiration. Fructose, however, did. They concluded, therefore, that "diabetes is associated with a defect in intracellular carbohydrate oxidation." In other words, it's not the sugar that causes diabetes, but rather impaired cellular respiration, *and fructose from natural foods may be beneficial.* These findings are, of course, in alignment with the previously mentioned reports.

Many anti-sugarists claim that fructose is poorly absorbed and that the liver limits how much can be absorbed. However, studies that actually monitor fructose metabolism have demonstrated that when fructose is consumed along with glucose (as is *always* the case with natural food sources), absorption is dramatically increased,[19] nullifying these claims of the anti-sugarists.

Yet another (false) sensationalistic claim made against fructose is that it is metabolized in the same way that alcohol is. Since it is widely accepted that alcohol is harmful for health (and for good reason, I might add), this charge seeks to make fructose guilty by association. But the claim is utter nonsense. Alcohol is a toxin that is first broken down into acetaldehyde, which is a toxin and probable carcinogen. Acetaldehyde is then converted to acetic acid, which is essentially non-toxic. However, the capacity of the

[18] Simonson et al. Normalization of carbohydrate-induced thermogenesis by fructose in insulin-resistant states. American Journal of Physiology. 1988; 254(2 pt 1): E201-E207.

[19] Sun SZ and Empie MW. Fructose metabolism in humans - what isotopic tracer studies show us. Nutrition and Metabolism. 2012; 9: 89.

body to make that conversion is easily overwhelmed. That is why small amounts of alcohol are generally not problematic, but anything more than very small amounts produces liver damage, brain damage, and general injury to the body.

Fructose, on the other hand, is metabolized differently. As previously mentioned, it is converted eventually to glucose, lactate, glycogen, carbon dioxide, and palmitic acid, none of which are toxic in the amounts produced. And, furthermore, none of the intermediate steps in the process produce any toxins. The metabolism of fructose is completely different than that of alcohol, and the claims that they are the same are ignorant or disingenuous. In fact, ironically, it turns out that fructose increases the rate at which alcohol is metabolized, decreasing the toxicity![20]

Finally, admittedly, there are a *few* studies (which I have cited in earlier works) that demonstrate that frequent consumption of large amounts of soda (one liter or more a day) can produce some subtle but slightly ominous indications in human health. Anti-sugarists are often quick to claim that it is the *fructose* in the soda that causes these problems. But first of all, these studies do *not* prove causation, and the noted changes are far from dramatic. Secondly, it's a heck of a leap to jump from the results of the studies to the claim that fructose is causing health problems. We really have to put this all into perspective.

Reportedly, the high-fructose corn syrup used in sodas may be slightly higher in fructose than glucose, but not dramatically (HFCS 55, used in soda, is 55 percent fructose and 42 percent glucose). And numerous studies have demonstrated that high-fructose corn syrup (even HFCS 55) is metabolized almost identically to sucrose in the human body. Meanwhile, sucrose feeding studies tend to demonstrate that sucrose is fairly benign. So is it really *fructose* that is to blame for the results of excessive soda consumption? Or might it be, I don't know...soda?

---

[20] Mascord et al. The effect of fructose on alcohol metabolism and on the [lactate]/[pyruvate] ratio in man. Alcohol and Alcoholism. 1991; 26(1): 53-59.

Sometimes we've just got to tell the truth about things. Soda is not synonymous with fructose, and so if some symptoms arise sometimes in connection with regular soda consumption, maybe it's the *soda* that causes the symptoms and not fructose.

At the end of the day, given the findings in the literature in regard to fructose, it seems to me that fructose is benign and likely even healthful *when consumed as part of a natural food*. That includes, by the way, white sugar, (sucrose), which is a natural, even if refined, food. I'm cautious about high-fructose corn syrup, to be honest, simply because it is a *highly* processed, industrial product that is not time-tested (which doesn't necessarily make it bad, but it doesn't lend much in the way of warm and fuzzy feelings either), and because the studies on high-fructose corn syrup show some mixed results. It is nothing dramatic, but there is still reason to be cautious. High-fructose corn syrup may be entirely benign, but I suspect that it is often contaminated with traces of heavy metals such as mercury,[21] which may account for some of the potential negative effects.

In any case, what seems to be the case with fructose is that anti-sugarists have cried wolf. There really doesn't seem to be any credible evidence that fructose is harmful *when it comes from real food* (which, again, includes white sugar, honey, maple syrup, and so forth). When study participants receive 35 percent of their energy intake from industrially produced free fructose, they experience health problems, and when study participants drink large amounts of soda made with high-fructose corn syrup, they may experience some minor, potentially negative effects. But neither of those demonstrates that fructose from natural foods in the amounts that people actually eat is actually problematic. In fact, there is substantial evidence suggesting quite the opposite; even high intake of fructose from real food is generally associated with good health.

---

[21] Bose-O'Reilly et al. Mercury exposure and children's health. Current problems in pediatric and adolescent health care. 2010; 40(8): 186-215.

Does Sugar Make Us Fat?

Sugar is said to make people fat. Nancy Appleton says so, Dr. Mark Hyman says so, Dr. Joe Mercola says so, and so do the rest of the anti-sugarists. But is it true? Well, interestingly, it turns out that *exactly the opposite* has been found in studies. There appears to be an *inverse* relationship in that the more sugar people consume, the less fat they tend to be. This finding has been reported time and time again. For example, researchers from the University of Dundee in Scotland studied over 11,000 people and found that the trimmer people ate substantially more sugar than the fatter people.[22] A study performed at the University of Leeds examined national survey data and found that sugar consumption did not correlate to body mass index (BMI) in women whereas higher sugar consumption correlated to *lower* BMI in men.[23] A New Zealand study found that low sugar consumption was associated with increased fatness whereas high sugar consumption was associated with leanness.[24] Need I really go on?

---

[22] Bolton-Smith C and Woodward M. Dietary composition and fat to sugar ratios in relation to obesity. International Journal of Obesity and Related Metabolic Disorders. 1994; 18(12): 820-828.

[23] Macdiarmid et al. The sugar-fat relationship revisited. International Journal of Obesity and Related Metabolic Disorders. 1998; 22(11): 1053-1061.

[24] Parnell et al. Exploring the relationship between sugar and obesity. Public Health Nutrition. 2008; 11(8): 860-866.

The results are fairly universally similar; sugar consumption is *not* linked to fatness.

High-fructose corn syrup (HFCS) has *not* been proven to be a significant cause in the overall trend toward increased fatness among the human population, either. A recent review of available studies examining the effects of HFCS on children determined that there is "inconclusive evidence definitively linking HFCS to obesity in children."[25] In other words, the potential link hasn't been *dis*proven, but neither is the evidence conclusive in favor of the theory.

Another review of studies looking at the link between HFCS and weight gain among the entire population also found no conclusive causal link. The authors concluded that "HFCS does not appear to contribute to overweight and obesity any differently than do other energy sources."[26]

The theory that HFCS causes people to become fat was put forward in a 2004 paper published in the *American Journal of Clinical Nutrition* by Bray et al. That paper presented the hypothesis that HFCS may have been the cause of American weight gain from 1970 to 2000. During that time, BMI (which is used as the primary determinant of obesity for statistical purposes) increased substantially in the United States. Meanwhile, consumption of HFCS increased by tenfold. The theory is certainly based on an interesting observation. But further examination has disproven it thoroughly. (Interestingly, consumption of polyunsaturated seed oils also increased during that same time period.)

According to the US Department of Agriculture Economic Research Service, US sugar consumption from both HFCS *and* sucrose peaked in 1999 and has been in decline since. And yet,

---

[25] Morgan RE. Does consumption of high-fructose corn syrup beverages cause obesity in children? Pediatric Obesity. 2013; 8(4): 249-254.

[26] Forshee et al. A critical examination of the evidence relating high fructose corn syrup and weight gain. Critical reviews in food, science, and nutrition. 2007; 47(6): 561-582.

according to the national data, Americans continue to get fatter with each passing year. If HFCS was responsible for making people fatter, we would expect that with the decline in HFCS consumption there would be a concurrent decline in fatness, which is not the case.

It *is* true that a rat study showed that rats fed HFCS gained more weight than did rats fed equivalent amounts of sucrose. But these results have not been replicated in humans. So thus far, in humans, when it comes to weight gain, HFCS gets a pass. As noted earlier, I'm cautious about advocating for HFCS consumption because there is some evidence that it may sometimes be contaminated with heavy metals. And as an industrial product, I think it is in a different category than natural food, including natural sugars. But there just isn't any evidence to link it to weight gain in humans.

Years ago, dietary fat was blamed for making people fatter. Sugar is just the scapegoat du jour, but it is no more culpable than dietary fat was. As demonstrated in my book *Big Fat Lies*, the so-called "obesity epidemic" really isn't as simple as it's often made out to be. It's unlikely that people are getting fatter due to a single cause. Likely contributing factors for the ballooning waistlines include increased stress, lack of sleep, environmental chemical exposure, and pharmaceutical drug use. But sugar isn't among those factors. There isn't any credible link between sugar and fat gain. In fact, as we've seen, if there is any link whatsoever, natural sugar consumption appears to be linked to greater *leanness*.

Attention Deficit Hyperactivity Disorder

One of the most popular beliefs about sugar is that it causes attention deficit hyperactivity disorder (ADHD). This belief is so popular and so strongly held by many that I have no delusions that this book is likely to do much to dislodge the belief. But be that as it may, I will simply present to you the findings of more than three decades of research into the matter.

In the 1980s, a number of studies emerged that looked specifically at the effects of diet on hyperactivity. Among the studies, quite a few investigated the effects of *sugar* on hyperactivity. Despite the popular theory, none of the studies turned up any convincing evidence that sugar produced hyperactivity. In fact, to the contrary, a number of them actually showed a slight *improvement* in attention after participants ate sugar.

In 1995, a research team from Vanderbilt University performed a meta-analysis of the published studies that looked at the effects of sugar on hyperactivity.[27] The team looked only at well-designed studies that were double blind and used a placebo.

---

[27] Wolraich et al. The effect of sugar on behavior or cognition in children: a meta-analysis. Journal of the American Medical Association. 1995; 274(20): 1617-1621.

The authors concluded that "sugar does not affect the behavior or cognitive performance of children."

A study conducted by a pair of New York researchers[28] sought to determine whether sugar has any effect on aggression or attention in children. The researchers noted that "[c]ontrolled studies have failed to confirm any effect on hyperactivity," and so hyperactivity was not of interest to them in their study. What they found was that sugar had absolutely no effect on aggression. Nor did it have any effect on attention in those children who were considered to be normal. The only effect noted was a slight increase in inattentiveness among those who were diagnosed with attention deficit disorder. The authors note that the "result may be of questionable clinical significance." They also suggest that the result may be due to confounding factors in the study, and they suggest that the results should be replicated before any recommendations can be made. The results have not been replicated to date. In fact, a later publication concluded, upon reviewing the evidence, that the well-designed studies "failed to provide any evidence that sugar ingestion leads to untoward behavior in children with [ADHD] or in normal children."[29]

A Korean team looked at the matter in a slightly novel way.[30] They questioned whether sugar consumption led to the *development* of ADHD. They studied 107 children who were classified as being at high risk for developing ADHD and looked to see whether or not sugar consumption was a predictor of which children would be later diagnosed with the disorder. What they found was that total sugar intake was not a predictor. Instead, they found that those children who had low intake of

[28] Wender EH and Solanto MV. Effects of sugar on aggressive and inattentive behavior in children with attention deficit disorder with hyperactivity and normal children. Pediatrics. 1991; 88(5): 960-966.

[29] Krummel et al. Hyperactivity: is candy causal? Critical reviews in food science and nutrition. 1996; 36(1-2): 31-47.

[30] Kim Y and Chang H. Correlation between attention deficit hyperactivity disorder and sugar consumption, quality of diet, and dietary behaviors in school children. Nutrition Research and Practice. 2011; 5(3): 236-245.

vitamin C and those children who obtained their sugar primarily from refined sources were at higher risk. In other words, a diet that is deficient in nutrients (aside from sugar that is) predicts the risk of being diagnosed with ADHD. The researchers did not consider whether nutritional quality of the children's diets was a stand-in for other factors such as economic status, so we don't know whether nutritional status is likely to be a cause or not. But in any case, sugar was not implicated.

Recently, a group of medical doctors and PhDs published a paper proposing a different mechanism by which sugar might cause ADHD.[31] The lead author of the paper is a man named Richard Johnson, MD, of the University of Colorado. By the authors' own admission, no convincing link between sugar and ADHD has yet been found. And, in fact, they admit that the research to date has largely disproven the leading theories proposing a connection. However, the authors suggest that a link may exist that hasn't been found yet. It seems to me that they are grasping at straws. They propose that perhaps chronic sugar consumption is a predictor of the development of ADHD, but as previously mentioned, the Korean researchers have shown that to be unlikely. The authors suggest that a link is likely to exist because sugar intake and ADHD are both associated with increased fatness. Yet the authors fail to provide a single citation to back their claim that sugar intake is associated with fatness. As noted, it's not.

The final argument that Johnson et al. make is based on the observation that sugar consumption increases dopamine concentrations in rats. The authors then postulate that sugar consumption may similarly create dopamine surges in humans, leading to ADHD. Unfortunately, this last argument, though certainly novel and interesting, is too much of a stretch to be believable. We have been told that dopamine is a neurotransmitter that causes a feeling of pleasure and is involved

---

[31] Johnson et al. Attention-deficit/hyperactivity disorder: is it time to reappraise the role of sugar consumption? Postgraduate Medical Journal. 2011; 123(5): 39-49;

in drug addiction. So when authors suggest that sugar may increase dopamine, it may not seem like such a leap to suggest that sugar may be the cause of ADHD. But let's consider some other activities that increase dopamine concentrations. Among them are reading, exercise, sex, listening to music, eating *any* enjoyable food, and a really good date. Oh, and get this: Increases in dopamine actually *increase attention*. And a Vanderbilt team found that humans considered to be go-getters have higher levels of dopamine than slackers.[32]

So the mere fact that sugar consumption may temporarily increase dopamine levels in the brain does not actually suggest *anything* about sugar except that there is a likelihood that sugar consumption was perceived as rewarding in those cases. It *is* true that, in extreme cases, *binges* of various substances ranging from opiates to alcohol to pornography to gambling to exercise to fatty- and/or carbohydrate-rich food can apparently down-regulate dopamine receptors. In other words, dopamine sensitivity can become blunted. And that may have negative consequences. But the key is that those changes occur with *binges*. Plenty of people drink small amounts of alcohol regularly without problems. Plenty of people are capable of playing a slot machine once or twice just for fun and then walking away. Plenty of people are able to eat a piece of cake for dessert and be satisfied. *Anything* could blunt dopamine sensitivity if done in great excess, but that doesn't make everything inherently problematic.

Interestingly, however, the rat studies that demonstrated "addiction-like responses" in response to sugar (glucose) were specifically designed to produce such responses. One such study[33] looked at the differences between two groups of rats. One group had full-time access to both rat chow and sugar water. The

---

[32] Treadway et al. Dopaminergic mechanism of individual differences in human effort-based decision making. Journal of Neuroscience. 2012; 32(18): 6170-6176.

[33] Avena et al. Evidence for sugar addiction: behavioral and neurochemical effects of intermittent, excessive sugar intake. Neuroscience and biobehavioral reviews. 2008; 32(1): 20-39.

other group was fasted for twelve hours a day and then given access to rat chow and sugar water. The researchers found that both groups ate the same amount. However, the rats that were deprived for twelve hours would "binge" on the sugar water during the first hour in which they were given access. I don't know about you, but that sounds like those poor rats were made to feel anxious that they might not have access to food again soon (which was true) and, as a result, they (sensibly) ate as much as they could of the most energy-dense option available as soon as they had access.

Unfortunately, the anxiety and bingeing behaviors that the researchers subjected these rats to created negative changes in the rats' dopamine sensitivity. The researchers then concluded that sugar must be just as addictive and harmful as cocaine, and later researchers like Johnson et al. decide that is evidence that sugar causes ADHD. But really, it's not. All it is evidence of is that, by depriving rats of food for half the day, it is possible to create unhealthy habits. Well, it also demonstrates that those who use animals in laboratories have deficient consciences. But that's another subject entirely.

Of course, regardless of the evidence to the contrary, plenty of parents still insist that feeding their kids concentrated sugar, whether that's candy or fruit juice, causes the kids to bounce off the walls. Researchers have investigated this as well. In what I consider to be a fairly brilliant study, a research team investigated whether reported effects of sugar on children are objectively true or if they are due to the expectations of the parents. In the study, five- to seven-year-old boys and their mothers were randomly placed into two groups. One group of mothers was told that their sons were given sugar. The other group was told that their sons were given a placebo. In fact, *all* the boys were given a placebo. None were given sugar.

The researchers then monitored the behavior of the children and the mothers. They also asked the mothers to describe their children's behavior. The mothers told their children were given sugar rated their children's behavior as "significantly more hyperactive" than the other mothers. The researchers also observed that the mothers in the sugar group "exercised more control by maintaining physical closeness, as well as showing trends to criticize, look at, and talk to their sons more than the control mothers."

I still don't expect most people will believe it's not the sugar, but there really isn't any evidence to support that theory. And if we can learn anything from those poor rats, it might be that placing restrictions only serves to increase the potential for unhealthy bingeing and negative changes in the brain.

Immunity

Search the Internet for the evils of sugar or have a five-minute conversation with your sugar-free zealot friend and you're almost guaranteed to hear the argument that sugar weakens immunity. This is yet another one of those attention-grabbing memes that is sure to persist for a long time. It doesn't matter if it's true; it just *sounds* so darn important.

But the trouble is that there's simply no proof that it is true. Of course the anti-sugar propagandists will often provide a reference for their claim. Almost invariably, the reference will be a 1973 paper published in the *American Journal of Clinical Nutrition*. The paper, titled *Role of sugars in human neutrophilic phagocytosis,*[34] doesn't actually show that sugar reduces immune function, despite the popular opinion to the contrary.

Here's what the paper is about: Some researchers gathered a group of eighteen human participants. The participants fasted overnight for twelve hours. In the morning, the participants were fed 100 grams of one of the following carbohydrates: glucose, starch, fructose, sucrose, honey, or orange juice. Blood was drawn from each of the participants at the following intervals: just prior to breaking the fast, as well as thirty minutes, one hour,

---

[34] Sanchez et al. Role of sugars in human neutrophilic phagocytosis. American Journal of Clinical Nutrition. 1973; 26(11): 1180-1184.

two hours, three hours, and five hours after eating the carbohydrate. Each time blood was drawn, it was mixed with a small amount of a pathogenic bacteria. The researchers then waited for half an hour and looked at the blood samples under a microscope. Tiny cells called phagocytes naturally occur in the blood and are part of the immune system. They "eat" pathogens, enveloping them. The researchers counted how many of the pathogenic bacteria each of the phagocytes had "eaten." This number is called the phagocytic index.

What the researchers found was that the phagocytic index changed after eating carbohydrates in all of the groups. In all groups, the fasting phagocytic index was approximately 16. In the starch group, the phagocytic index rose to 17.7 half an hour after eating and then dropped to 14.4 at one hour and all the way down to 13.6 at the five-hour mark. In contrast, the honey group held constant from fasting to the 30-minute mark but then dropped to 9.7 and didn't increase again until the three-hour mark when the phagocytic index reached 12.4. The other groups followed a similar pattern, dropping to about 13 at the half hour mark, continuing to drop for another hour or two, and then slowly increasing up to the five-hour mark.

Now this is certainly an interesting study, but it doesn't provide any conclusive evidence that sugar harms immune health. In fact, the study asks far more questions than it answers. The authors don't try to draw any conclusions, and at the end of the paper, they make it clear that the study is only scratching the surface of an interesting field of study. The *only* aim of the study was to measure the effects of different carbohydrates on phagocytic index, but the *significance* of that is not clear to the researchers or the readers. And if a lower phagocytic index is worse than a higher index, the natural conclusion that could be drawn from the study would be that it is best not to eat at all, or at least not to eat any carbohydrates, which is a very bad idea. So I really don't recommend doing that. And keep in mind that this single, inconclusive, possibly irrelevant study merely measures the phagocytic index of *drawn blood*. We don't know what the effects are in a living human.

Based on this one study, we have no idea what to make of the results. The authors note additional investigations into the effects of protein and dietary fats on phagocytosis. However, I have not been able to find another study published by any of the authors with any reference to phagocytosis. I *have* found a handful of equally inconclusive (and often even less relevant) studies published by other authors that look at the effects of dietary alterations on phagocytosis; it is mostly about the effects of different types of dietary fats. However, I haven't found a single study that demonstrates what the findings mean.

Although no experiments have been done on live humans to determine the actual effects of dietary sugar on immune function, a number of studies strongly contradict the claim that sugar harms immunity. Three studies found that sugar in blood actually *increased* the rate at which bacteria were removed through phagocytosis.[35] It was also found that while artificial sweeteners did not do anything to improve immunity, natural sweeteners modulated the immune response. Natural sweeteners increased the immune response in blood infected with pathogens, but they produced no increase in immune response in healthy blood. And other researchers found that rats fed honey or sucrose *increased* phagocytosis compared to rats fed sugar-free diets.[36] Researchers

---

[35] Mesaik et al. Honey modulates oxidative burst of professional phagocytes. Phytotherapy Research. 2008; 22(10): 1404-1408; Rahiman F and Pool EJ. The effects of Saccharum officinarum (sugar cane) molasses on cytokine secretion by human blood cultures. Journal of Immunoassay and Immunochemistry. 2010; 31(2): 148-159;

Rahiman F and Pool EJ. The in vitro effects of artificial and natural sweeteners on the immune system using whole blood culture assays. Journal of Immunoassay and Immunochemistry. 2014; 35(1): 26-36.

[36] Chepulis LM. The effects of honey compared with sucrose and a sugar-free diet on neutrophil phagocytosis and lymphocyte numbers after long-term feeding in rats. Journal of Complementary and Integrative Medicine. 2007; 4(1): 1-7.

have also found that sugarcane juice improves immunity in chickens.[37]

We also know that many types of sugar have been traditionally valued for *boosting* immune health. Many of us may know of honey's traditional use as an immune enhancer, and we probably know of various folk remedies that use honey to treat a cold. In India's traditional healing system Ayurveda, dried sugarcane juice, called jaggery, is used and valued for its health-promoting properties and has been for *thousands of years*. It is used along with honey and a long list of herbs in a traditional jam called chyawanprash, which is used regularly to strengthen immunity. Other Ayurvedic traditional remedies also make use of jaggery to increase immune health. And in North America, maple sap, which is boiled down to syrup, has long been enjoyed as a spring tonic, believed to increase health and vitality.

Science is now starting to confirm some of these traditional uses. So even those who scoff at folk remedies now have reason to take notice that natural sugars may, in fact, improve immunity. The research is very preliminary, but it confirms precisely what many people have known for a long time. One study found that mice fed honey and injected with dead E. coli had a significantly stronger and more successful immune response than did mice fed a honey-free diet.[38] And a number of studies performed by a University of Rhode Island team have shown that maple syrup contains many novel compounds that are antibacterial and that

---

[37] Awais et al. Immunotherapeutic effects of some sugar cane extracts against coccidiosis in industrial broiler chickens. Experimental Parasitology. 2011; 128(2): 104-110.

El-Abasy et al. Preventative and therapeutic effects of sugar cane extract on cyclophosphamide-induced immunosuppression in chickens. International Immunopharmacology. 2004; 4(8): 983-990.

[38] Al-Waili NS and Haq A. Effect of honey on antibody production against thymus-dependent and thymus-independent antigens in primary and secondary immune response. Journal of Medicinal Food. 2004; 7(4): 491-494.

help to modulate the immune system.[39] Plus, lest we forget, study after study shows that fruit consumption is positively correlated with every aspect of health, including immune health.

So what has happened is that the ideological disdain for sugar has blinded people to the facts staring us plainly in the face. Natural sugars, *particularly* in their less processed state, have a long tradition for increasing health and immunity, and science largely confirms those traditional uses. But instead of reporting on that, what we have is a faulty conclusion drawn from a single study 40 years ago that is being repeated over and over again, further blinding people to the fact that it's just not true. Sugar isn't inherently harmful for immunity and may actually be helpful.

---

[39] Li L and Seeram NP. Maple syrup phytochemicals include lignans, coumarins, a stilbene, and other previously unreported antioxidant phenolic compounds. Journal of Agricultural and Food Chemistry. 2010; 58(22): 11673-11679; Li L and Seeram NP. Further investigation into maple syrup yields three new lignans, a new phenylpropanoid, and twenty-six other phytochemicals. Journal of Agricultural and Food Chemistry. 2011; 59(14): 7708-7716.

Teeth

Everyone knows that sugar causes dental cavities, right? Well, think again. It *is* true that *any* carbohydrates left in the mouth for long periods of time can *indirectly* contribute to tooth decay. However, sugar itself does not *cause* cavities.

How *do* dental cavities form? They form because of *acids* that erode the enamel and dentin layers of the tooth. Of course, swishing vinegar, lemon juice, or Coca-Cola (which contains phosphoric acid and has a pH of 2.5) in the mouth will erode the protective layers of the teeth. But most people aren't doing that. So the primary source of acids that erode teeth is the bacteria in the mouth.

Like the gut and the skin, the mouth contains a microbiome of bacteria.[40] Interestingly, recent trends in dental health have shown that oral probiotics can reverse early signs of decay and prevent further decay. A number of products are presently marketed specifically for this purpose. It turns out that by modifying the bacteria in the mouth, it is possible to prevent the formation of biofilms and acid production.

When the oral microbiome contains bacteria that form biofilms, the result is plaque on the teeth; it is a familiar

---

[40] Dewhirst et al. The human oral microbiome. Journal of Bacteriology. 2010; 192(19): 5002-5017.

phenomenon that most of us have been trained to deal with through brushing and flossing. The biofilm houses the bacteria colonies, which will use carbohydrates in the mouth as food. The end product of the bacterial digestion of carbohydrates is some type of acid. Since the biofilm coats the teeth, the acid tends to affect the teeth in particular.

However, when the bacteria that predominates in the oral microbiome are of a different sort, plaque will not form nor will tooth decay occur. Or, alternatively, if the mouth is routinely rinsed thoroughly after eating, carbohydrates will not remain in the mouth for acid-producing bacteria to convert to acids. Either way, no acids to contribute to decay. And either way, sugar is just fine.

However, the story isn't merely as simple as the microbiome. As noted in *How I Healed My Teeth While Eating Sugar*, teeth are living tissue and their health depends upon total nutrition and metabolic health. The health of teeth depends upon adequate energy, protein, minerals, and fat-soluble vitamins, among other things. Eliminating sugar will not prevent cavities if the diet is lacking in any of those factors and, on the flip side, as long as those factors are adequate, dietary sugar plays an extremely minor role in the potential for cavity formation. When nutrition is adequate, stress is low, sleep is good, and basic dental hygiene is followed (namely, rinsing the mouth at least once a day to reduce fermentable stuff in the mouth), the risk of dental cavities is low. And, in fact, I actually had an enormous cavity heal naturally while I was eating a pound of sugar daily. Again, that's merely an n=1 report, but it does refute the notion that sugar is the actual cause of cavities.

Candida

Of course, no discussion of sugar would be complete without a mention of *Candida albicans*, the bugaboo of alternative health subscribers. The anti-sugarists claim candida must be starved by eliminating all sugar from the diet. A quick consultation with Google returns 1.7 billion results for diets that seek to solve supposed candida problems by eliminating sugar. Recognizing that all digestible carbohydrates eventually turn into sugar (because that's what the body needs), many advocates of candida starvation protocols suggest that eliminating dietary sugar isn't enough. *All* carbohydrates have to be eliminated, from granulated sugar to bread to fruit to carrots.

What Google doesn't know, and what peer-reviewed papers in journals don't know, is what the success rate of those diets is in terms of eliminating candida overgrowth. I know of no formal study of the matter. It's not a question that's included in standard national surveys. So I can't give you any reliable statistics. But based on about 50 conversations I have had with people starving themselves—er, I mean, starving candida with a no sugar, no fruit, no potatoes, no bread, no pasta, no carrots diet—I'm fairly confident that the success rate is well under 1 percent.

There's good reason why these starvation protocols (starving candida, of course) are doomed to fail. The science behind them is deeply flawed. In the first place, studies have shown that feeding sugar does not cause *Candida albicans* overgrowth.[41] And based on everything covered thus far, it should be clear now that starving candida would be impossible without starving the human, at least if we're talking about a systemic overgrowth which is what most people seem to be convinced that they are dealing with. Here's why: If candida is in the blood (i.e., a systemic overgrowth), then it will *always* have a steady supply of sugar so long as the human is alive. Why? Because if blood sugar levels fall too low, it can be fatal. Normal fasting blood sugar levels are in the range of 70 to 80 mg/dl. If levels fall below 60, most people will feel lousy. If levels fall below 40, that can produce seizures. And below 10 results in coma and potentially death. It's worth repeating at this point that we *need* sugar to live. You can't starve candida. Don't try.

What does seem to be the case is that there is a connection between impaired cellular respiration and *Candida albicans* overgrowth. In fact, candida overgrowth is a common occurrence (medically diagnosed) in those with type 2 diabetes. This fact has led many anti-sugarists to proclaim that candida *causes* diabetes and that sugar *causes* candida overgrowth. But they may be putting the cart before the horse. There's no evidence that candida causes diabetes. Rather, the most likely explanation is that candida is an opportunistic organism (aren't we all) that tries to metabolize excess sugar in the blood in cases of insulin resistance (impaired cellular respiration). Looking at it that way, we could even argue that candida is *beneficial*.

If, in fact, the primary problem in systemic candida overgrowth is impaired cellular respiration, then the only successful way to address the problem is to address the root cause. Sugar is not the root cause. Impaired cellular respiration is, and that may be caused by any number of factors such as excessive linoleic acid in the diet, excessive stress, poor sleep

---

[41] Weig et al. Limited effect of refined carbohydrate dietary supplementation on colonization of the gastrointestinal tract of healthy subjects by Candida albicans. American Journal of Clinical Nutrition. 1999; 69(6): 1170-1173.

quality or duration, or excessive radiation exposure. Sugar doesn't make that list.

Exposing Some Good Sense

Pundits, politicians, medical professionals, and hucksters alike bombard us with their scaremongering. We're reminded often of the high rates of cardiovascular disease, diabetes, cancer, and other diseases, and we're encouraged and sometimes even mandated to reduce our risk. Amidst the hysteria, everyone is looking for something to blame. Sugar has become a scapegoat. In fact, sugar has been called "the new tobacco." However, the evidence against sugar is practically nonexistent.

Anti-sugarists have leveled an incredible number of accusations against sugar. In fact, Nancy Appleton, author of *Lick the Sugar Habit*, has "141 reasons sugar ruins your health" listed on her website. That's a lot of accusations. But it turns out that they are largely fabrications, myths, and lies. They are unsubstantiated claims.

What about all those people who say they feel better when they eliminate or greatly reduce sugar from their diets? Well, the problem is often that those reports are confounded by other variables. When people cut out sugar, they often cut out soda and fast food. The *quality* of the food they eat may improve completely independent of sugar. The simple fact that someone desires to make what he or she perceives to be positive changes in his or her life can account for positive outcomes either due to placebo effect or because of other positive changes made at the same time, such as making time for sleep or walking or loving relationships. Also, we rarely get follow-ups on testimonials, so we don't know what happens six months later. Anecdotally, from the few reports that I've read, the honeymoon phase wears off in the long run, and stress begins to increase with most extreme diets, including diets that seek to eliminate all sugar.

Hopefully, in reading this, you've begun to see that natural sugars of various sorts (like cane sugar, beet sugar, honey, maple syrup, fruit, and sweet vegetables) are *not* the cause of the many awful things blamed on them and may, in fact, have many *virtues*. First and foremost, of course, I hope that you've opened your mind to the fact that sugar is an essential element of human life whether we obtain it from dietary sugar, protein, or fat, or from our own muscles and organs in starvation states. If blood sugar drops too low, then *pfft!* Lights out.

That's just the beginning of the benefits of sugars. Sugars of all kinds have been used successfully in promoting wound healing for thousands of years. Honey is best known for this, and a number of studies have shown that honey has immunomodulating effects both internally (as stated earlier) as well as when applied topically to wounds.[42] Honey has even been used successfully to treat diabetic foot ulcers.[43] Although honey is more popular and more effective in the treatment of wounds, sucrose can also be used effectively.[44]

Various natural sugars are also effective antioxidants. Many disease states are linked to increased oxidative stress, so antioxidants help to improve health by reducing that stress. Fruits are notoriously loaded with antioxidants as well as sugar, and high fruit intake is strongly associated with good health. Various types

[42] Majtan J. Honey: an immunomodulator in wound healing. Wound Repair and Regeneration. 2014; 22(2): 187-192.

[43] Makhdoom et al. Management of diabetic foot by natural honey. Journal of Ayub Medical College. 2009; 21(1): 103-105.

[44] Mphande et al. Effects of honey and sugar dressings on wound healing. Journal of Wound Care. 2007; 16(7): 317-319.

of honey have been shown to have antioxidant activity.[45] The University of Rhode Island research team cited earlier has found maple syrup to have a large number of antioxidants. Sugarcane also has powerful antioxidant properties. It has been found to protect against radiation-induced damage.[46] Traditionally, the juice of the whole sugarcane plant has been used therapeutically, but research shows that the molasses is the part richest in antioxidants.[47]

Sugar in various forms has been valued both as food and medicine for thousands of years. In India, sugarcane has been used for as far back as anyone can remember, and for nearly 2500 years, it has been processed into crystallized sugar. In neighboring Nepal, rock paintings dated to 2500 years ago show that harvesting honey was of tremendous importance. Honey has traditionally made up a significant part of the diets of many people. In fact, honey is so important to some traditional people that it makes up an impressive 80 percent of their total calories during honey season each year.[48]

To be clear, I am not suggesting that a diet composed exclusively or even mostly of refined sugar is likely to be healthy in the long run, because it's not (though it can be therapeutic in the short term for those who are recovering from restriction or impaired sugar metabolism). However, the reason that it wouldn't be healthy is not because it would cause cancer or diabetes. Instead, it's just that a diet that is comprised mostly of refined sugar would probably be deficient in other necessary nutrients. Even refined sugar is just fine in the context of a

---

[45] Mandal MD and Mandal S. Honey: its medicinal properties and antibacterial activity. Asian Journal of Tropical Biomedicine. 2011; 1(2): 154-160.

[46] Kadam et al. Antioxidant activity in sugarcane juice and its protective role against radiation-induced DNA damage. Food Chemistry. 2008; 106(3): 1154-1160.

[47] Valli et al. Sugar cane and sugar beet molasses, antioxidant rich alternatives to refined sugar. Journal of Agricultural and Food Chemistry. 2012; 60: 12508-12515.

[48] Lee RB and Daly R. The Cambridge Encyclopedia of Hunters and Gatherers. Cambridge: Cambridge University Press, 1999.

nutrient-replete diet that includes fruits, vegetables, starches, dairy, eggs, meat, fish, and so forth. Less-processed sugars such as maple syrup, cane sugar with molasses intact, honey, and so forth might even be considered *health foods*.

Hopefully, the takeaway from this book has been that natural sugar is nothing to fear and may even offer unique health benefits in the right context. I'm certainly not suggesting that you start guzzling two-liter bottles of Coca-Cola and scarfing down Mars bars like they are going out of style. But a spoonful or two (or three) of natural sugar, refined or otherwise, in your coffee or tea or to sweeten some hot chocolate? What's the problem? A delicious drizzle of real maple syrup atop your waffle? Hey, it might just help protect against cancer![49] Some honey on your buttered toast? That could protect your stomach and increase your immunity. Some fruit or (gasp!) fruit *juice*? It's *good* for you.

---

[49] Gonzalez-Sarrias et al. Effects of maple plant part extracts on proliferation, apoptosis and cell cycle arrest of human tumorigenic and non-tumorigenic colon cells. Phytotherapy Research. 2012; 26(7): 995-1002.

Get Another of My Books for Free

If you've enjoyed this book, there's more where this one came from. And I'd be delighted to give you another one of my books (normally priced at $3.99) for free.

My book *Cleansed* is a reader favorite. Here are some of the things reviewers have to say about it:

> *"[G]et the book and enjoy Joey's gift of explaining and educating through the written word"*
>
> *"Finally, some sense"*
>
> *"This book was worth every minute I spent reading it."*
>
> *"I am so thankful to have found and read this book"*

Download your free digital copy of *Cleansed* today by visiting http://joeylotthealth.com/cleansed-free-offer

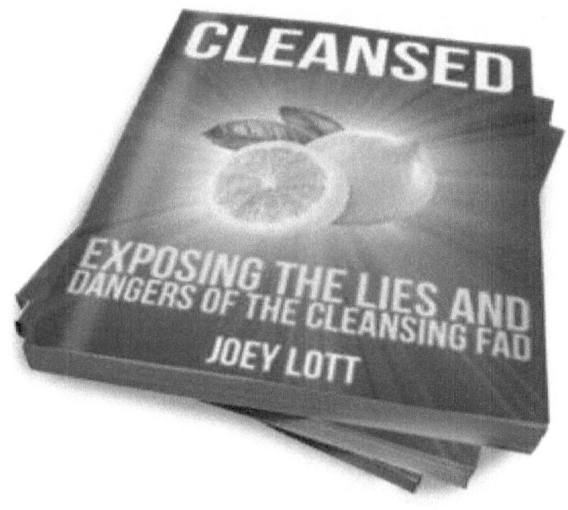

Please Write a Review of This Book

If you liked this book, it would be fabulous if you would write a review of it on site of the retailer from which you got the book

I know, I know. You think it doesn't matter. And it is sort of obnoxious that I ask you to take a minute from your valuable time to do something like write a review of this book.

But actually, reviews are really, really helpful. And that's the reason I ask.

See, the way the retailers work is they help potential readers to discover new books, *but only if those books have* recent *reviews*.

So if you liked this book and would like others to be able to discover it, please do take a moment right now to write a review and post it on the site of the retailer from which you got this book. It really does make a difference.

Thank you.

About the Author

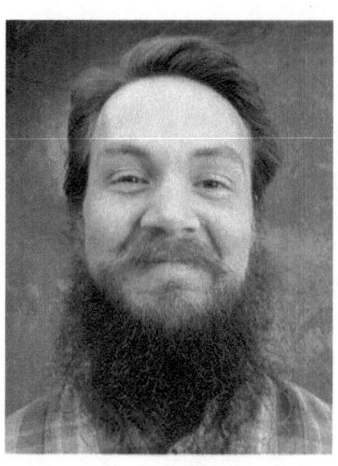

"Don't assume. Question. Look for yourself."
Joey Lott is a fresh and well-respected voice, and he has been described as "a real treasure".

He draws upon his own experiences and struggles, writing with a touch of authenticity and sincerity that is rare. He also draws upon a wealth of experience communicating with tens of thousands of people by phone and email to understand the struggles of others.

Lott lives in New Mexico, USA on a small homestead with his partner and children.

www.ingramcontent.com/pod-product-compliance
Lightning Source LLC
Chambersburg PA
CBHW050517290526
45786CB00007B/2606